Simplified

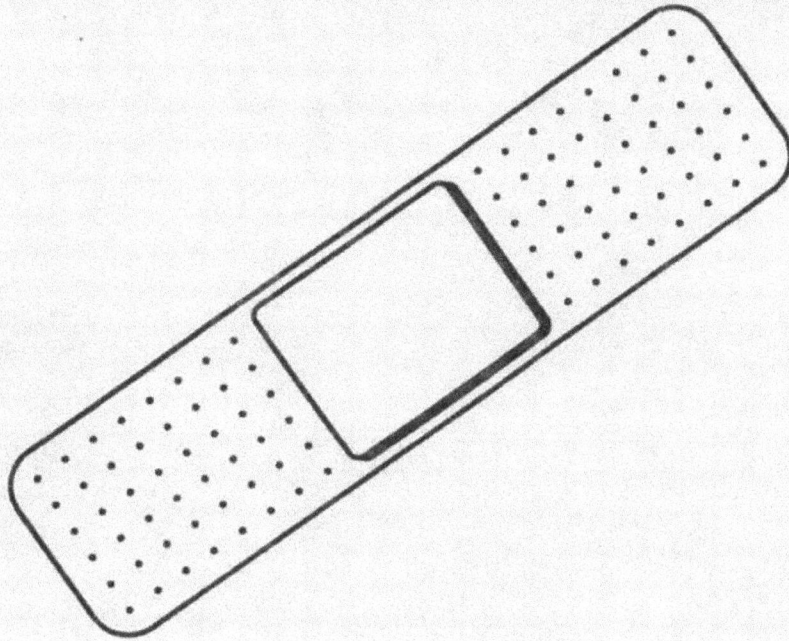

Clotting

By Malcom Rosenberg, R.N.

Simplified Clotting

Malcom Rosenberg
370 N.W. 115 Way
Coral Springs, FL 33071
(954) 753-5915

Copyrighted 2007
Printed in the United States of America

Blood an overview

An Adult has 5 to 6 liters of blood.

Blood flows through a network of arteries arterioles and veins on a circuit from the heart back to the heart. This series of pipes is about 60,000 miles long. Really. That is long enough to circle the Earth two times.

The most well known function of blood is to nourish all 6 trillions cells in the body. The red blood cells deliver oxygen and remove carbon dioxide.

To fight infection blood carries five types of white blood cells.

The next most appreciated job is clotting or hemostasis. This process limits blood loss from injuries.

IMPORTANT WORDS to RECOGNIZE
(You don't have to understand them yet.)

Part of the difficulty of learning clotting is that many of the important words sound very similar. I have grouped them by their similar sounds. There is no reason to define them here since they are mostly new. Just recognize that you will have to differentiate very similar words.

Thrombin
Prothrombin
Prothrombin time (PT)

Thrombus
thrombolytic

Fibrin
Fibrinogen
Fibrinolytic

Plasmin
plasminogen
Tissue plasimogen activator

Tissue thromboplastin
Partial thromboplastin time (PTT)

Hemostasis an overview

After an injury the body needs to stop the loss of blood. It does this by forming a clot at the site. That's obvious. It gets tricky because the body must know when to be liquid and when and where to turn solid. That is what this book is about.

This explanation of the clotting process will be broken down into three phases, (1) platelet aggregation, (2) clot formation and (3) clot lyseing.

PLATELETS

There are three steps in the clotting process, platelet aggregation, blood coagulation and clot dissolution. The first step (#1) in the process is platelet aggregation.

Platelets are the smallest particle in the blood.

There are about 1.5 trillion platelets in our body. More precisely: 1,497,458,253,769. The number of platelets per milliliter is in a complete blood count, a CBC. About 200 billion platletses are created each day. They live about nine days. 300,000 platelets in each milliliter is a normal count. You may have noticed platelet counts below 150,000 in the CBC. You may have hesitated to give an injection because of low platelet counts.

Normally platelets flow through the vasculature (all 60,000 miles of it) totally oblivious to each other or the lining of the vessels (smooth endothelial cells).

That is because platelets are normally repelled from each other and from the walls of the blood vessels. There are a few obvious reasons for this. One is the negative charge of the platelets. So the negatively charged bodies avoid each other.

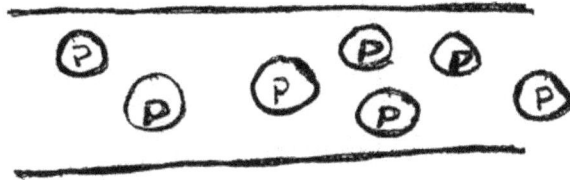

The other factor is smooth walls of the blood vessels. Nothing can stick to them. That is like the idea of Teflon pans. I don't know which came first. But it was a very good idea.

COLLAGEN

Just below the epithelial lining are very coarse collagen fibers. Just like your pots and pans, if you break the smooth Teflon lining, just below it is a very coarse surface. This is significant in the clotting process as we shall see. When there is an injury (a cut) which damages the endothelial lining platelets come into contact with these coarse collagen fibers.

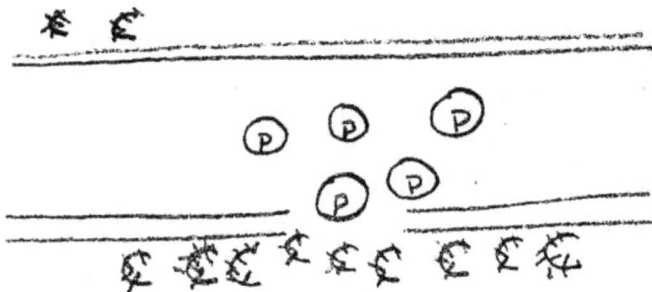

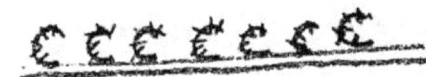

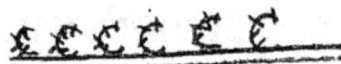

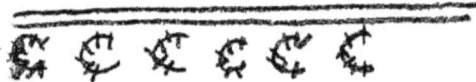

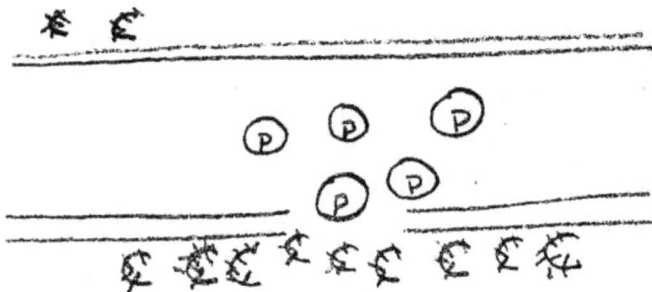

Say you cut yourself on you slicing potatoes and carrots.

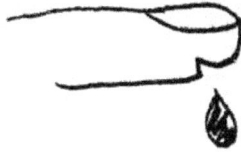

The injury causes a break in the nice smooth endothelial lining

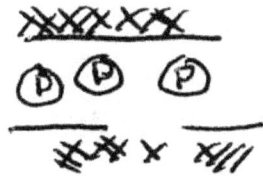

Platelets are attracted to the exposed collagen. They run to the collagen.

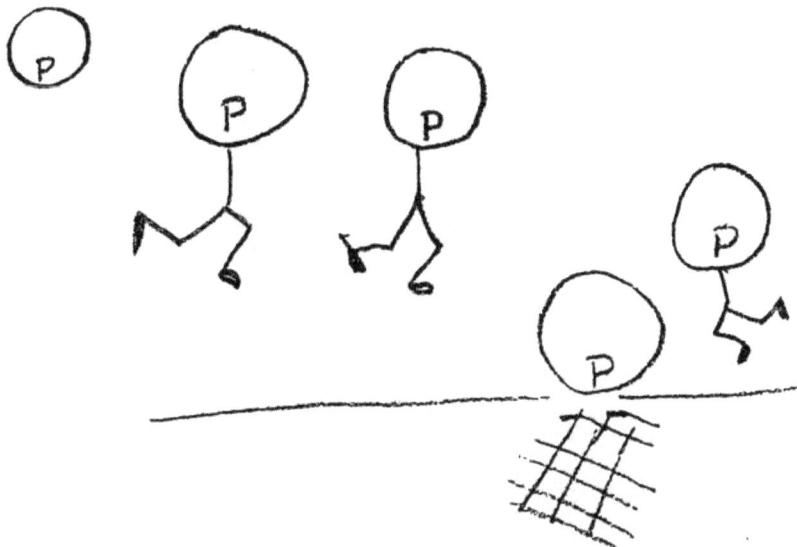

When platelets stick to the collagen, they change shape.

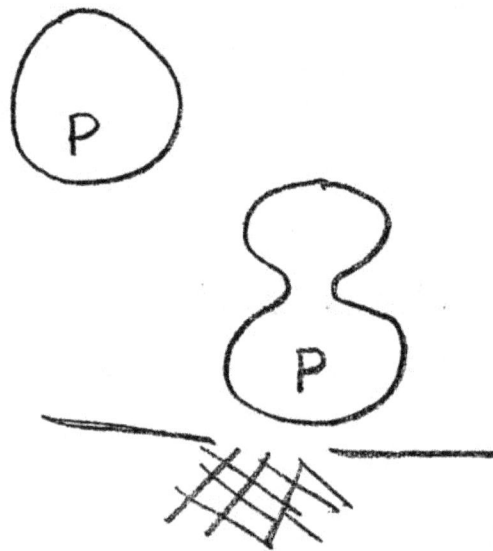

From this shape change the platelets degranulate or break apart. Chemicals called mediators leak out. They make the platelets sticky. Visualize these mediators as Elmer's Glue.

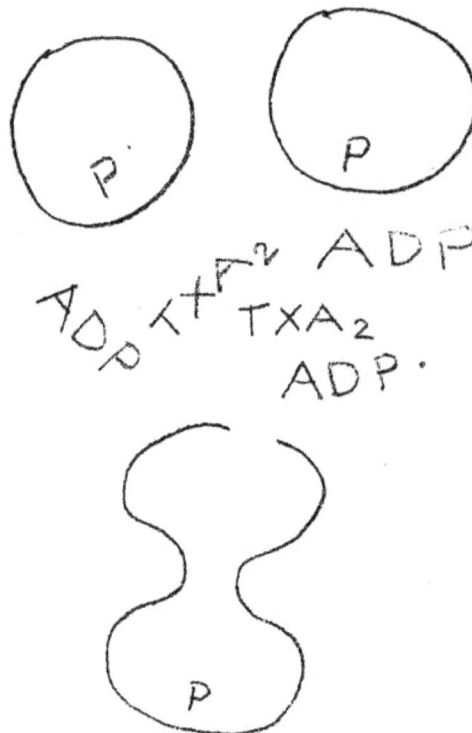

More specifically we are concerned with two mediators, adenosine Diphosphate (ADP) and thromboxane A_2. These mediators attract other platelets to the injury site

The newly arrived platelets adhere to already stuck platelets.

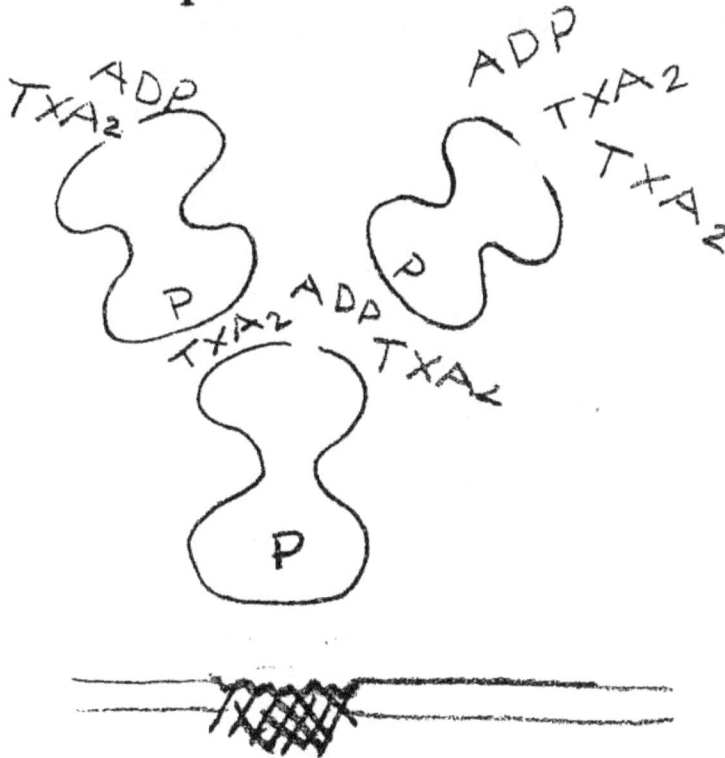

They change shape, break open, release more mediators, attract more platelets which adhere to......etc...etc.

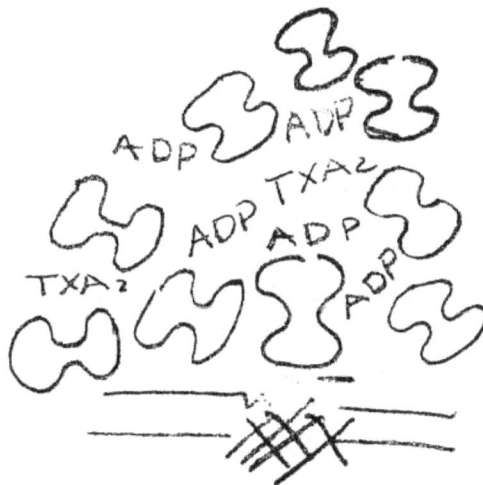

These broken (lysed) platelets quickly stop the bleeding This mass of platelets is called a thrombus. This process is called platelet adhesion.

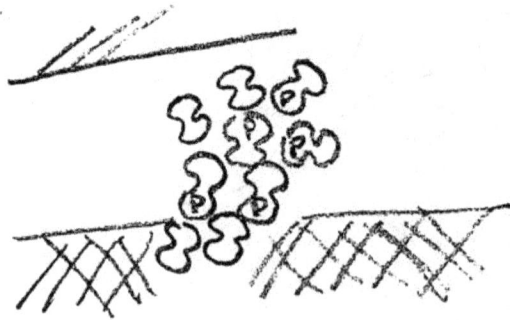

VASOCONSTRICTION

There is another hemostatic function that the mediators perform. Seretonin (a new one we haven't mentioned) and thromboxane A_2 cause the vessel to constrict. This is limited to smaller vessels. It would be more effective in a damaged capillary of your index finger than it would be in a ruptured aorta.

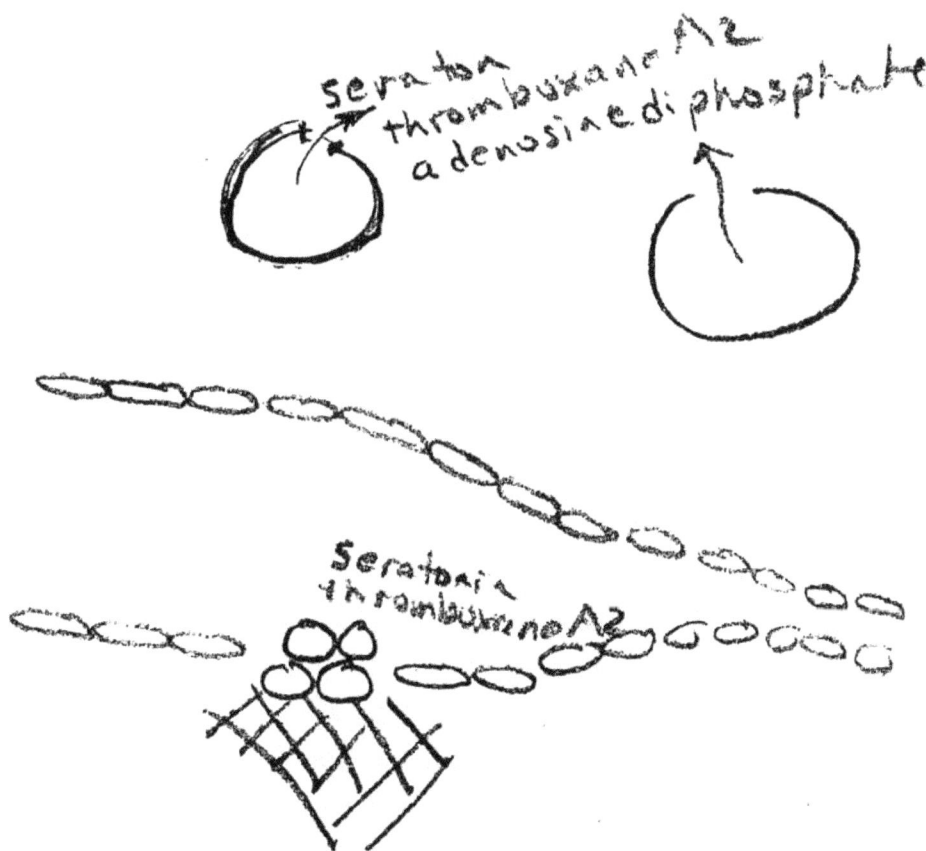

Enough Platelet Aggregation Already!

Like I said: The body must know when the blood should be liquid and when and where to be solid. If that process described above did not have some limits, we would turn into one big platelet aggregate every time we nicked our finger. What stops that runaway clot? Who you gonna call? Prostacyclin.

Prostacyclin (PGI_2) inhibits the release of aggregating agents, serotonin and thromboxane A_2 from the aggregating platelets. You can visualize prostacyclin as a cork in opening of the ruptured platelet. The healthy epithelial cells surrounding the injury secrete PGI_2.

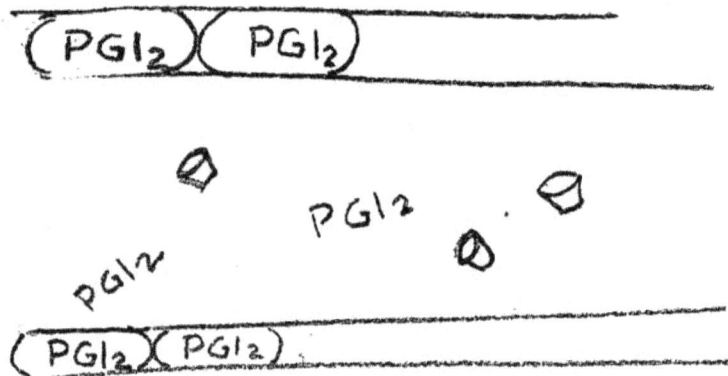

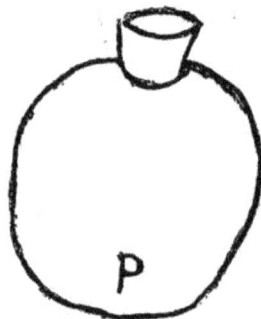

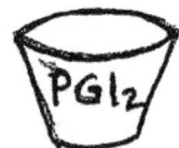

von Willebrand factor

The platelets are able to stick to the exposed collagen because of a coating called von Willebrand factor. Low levels of von Willebrand factor leaves platelets unable to adhere to the exposed collagen, or unable to form a platelet plug.

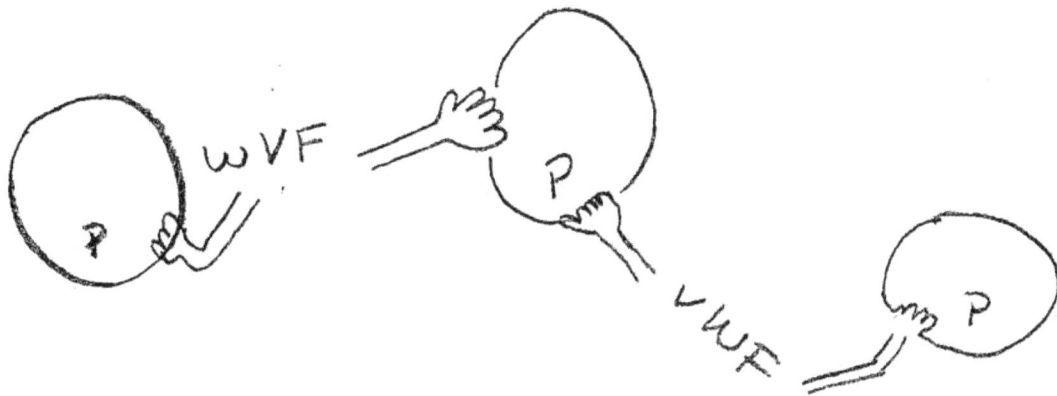

GPIIb/IIIa

That is the name of a platelet to platelet connector that plays a part in platelet aggregation, platelet glycoprotein IIb/IIIa. The picture explains this pretty well. ReoPro and Integrilin are used to prevent platelet aggregation. They are called platelet GPIIb/IIIa inhibitors. Who came up with that name Geepeetoobeethreeay?

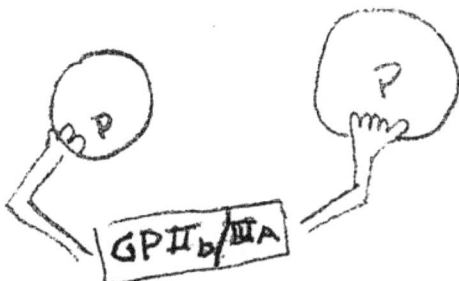

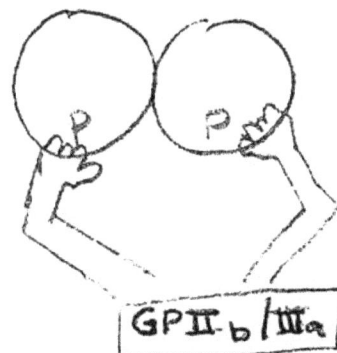

Drugs Platelet Aggregation Inhibitors

Do you remember (about two pages ago) that platelets release chemical mediators which attract floating platelets to the injury?

TXA2 ADP ADP TXA2

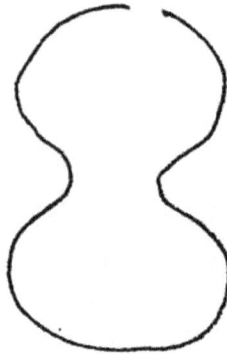

Platelet aggregation inhibitors (like aspirin) block those mediators.

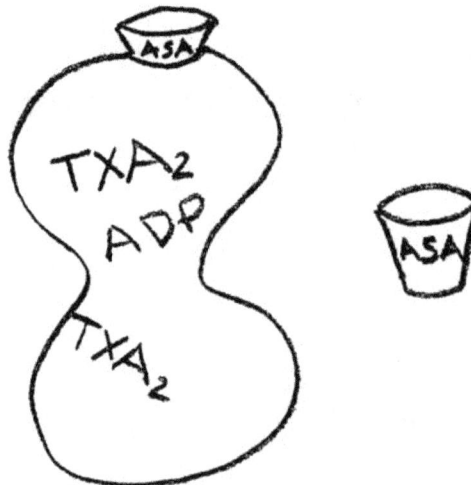

ASA

TXA$_2$ ADP TXA$_2$

ASA

Persantine potentiates prostacyclin (PGI$_2$) to decrease platelet adhesion mediators.

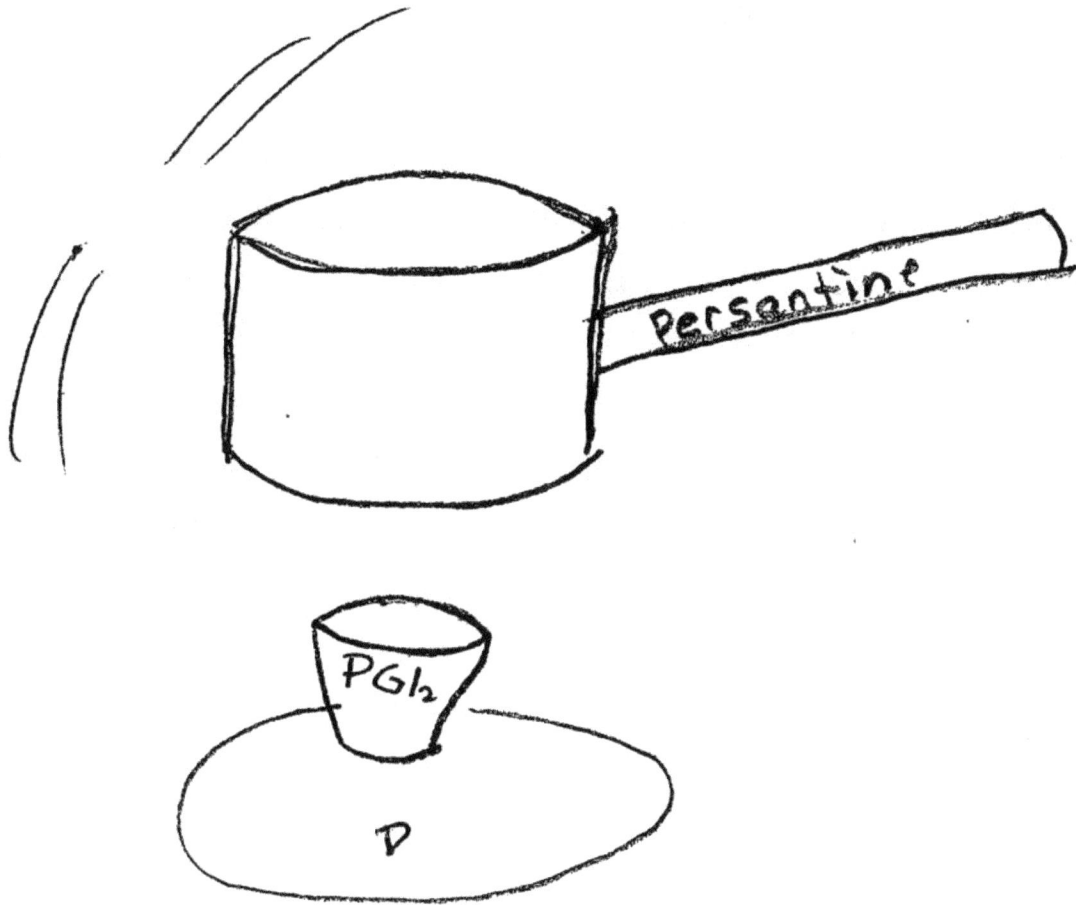

These lysed (broken) platelets quickly stop the bleeding. This sticky mass of platelets is called a thrombus. Up to this point the process is called platelet adhesion.

Next…….. **Clotting**…….tah duh

A platelet plug is a good start. It isn't strong enough. The injury needs a blood clot to provide good protection from bleeding. You know what blood clot looks like. It looks like a scab. Scab is medical terminology for a fibrin (you'll find out what that is) mesh which traps platelets and red blood cells. This is sort of like a sewer grate that gets covered with branches and leaves, then all the cans and plastic bottles, general litter, food wrappers and street debris totally clogs it. The next time you walk by a clogged up sewer think fibrin mesh.

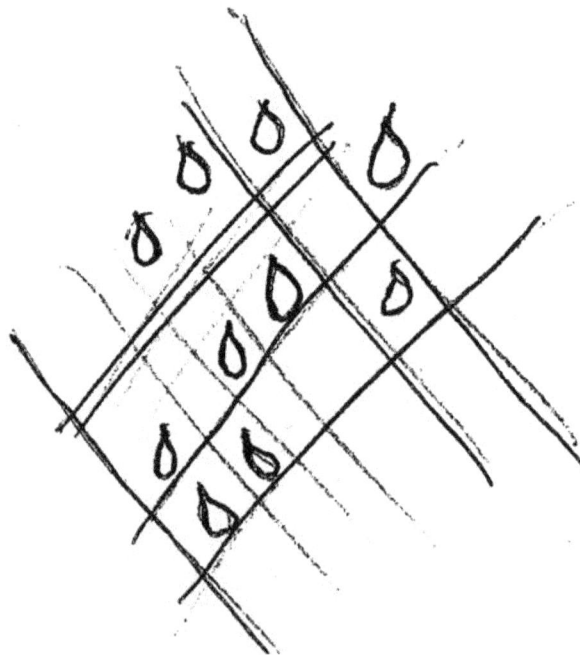

The clotting process is a series of steps. I have shown these as a row of dominoes. The first domino to fall is the injury. The last is the formation of the fibrin mesh.

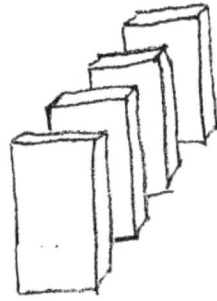

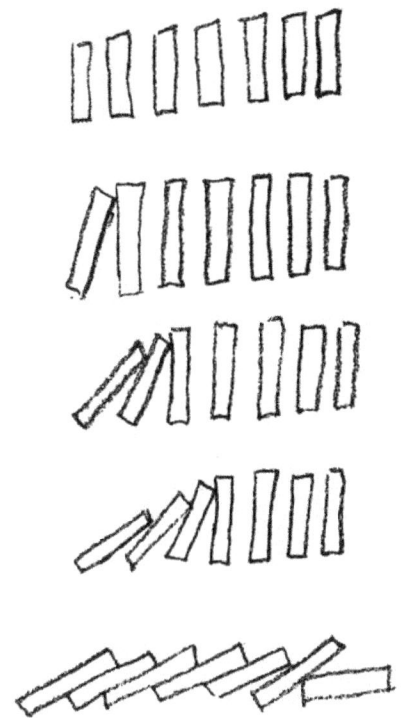

Blood clots by a sequential order of chemical reactions by so called clotting factors floating around in the blood. There are 12 clotting factors floating around in the blood. They are named by Roman Numerals, I, II, III, IV, V......X, XI, XII. They are not named in their order of activation. The injury activates the first clotting factor, which activates the next clotting factor until many steps later fibrinogen turns into fibrin which is a clot. This process is called the clotting cascade because it is like a series of water falls where each water fall collects in a pool which forms a larger waterfall than the previous one each step activates a stronger more vigorous water fall. In the next picture I have shown this as sequentially larger dominos.

The last three dominoes to fall are the activation of factor X, the conversion of thrombin to thrombin and the conversion of fibrinogen to fibrin (the clot). You should learn these names. They will reappear. Trust me.

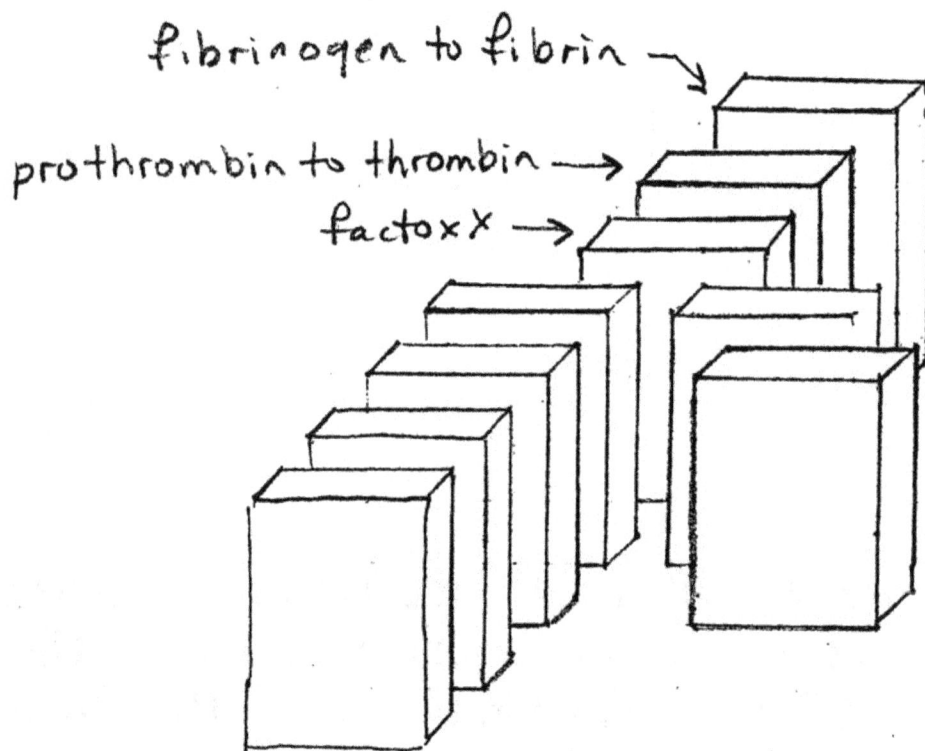

fibrinogen to fibrin →

prothrombin to thrombin →

factoxX →

EXTRINSIC AND INTRINSIC PATHWAYS

The single row of dominoes is not entirely accurate.

A Y- shaped row of dominoes is more accurate. This is how we will show the coagulation cascade.

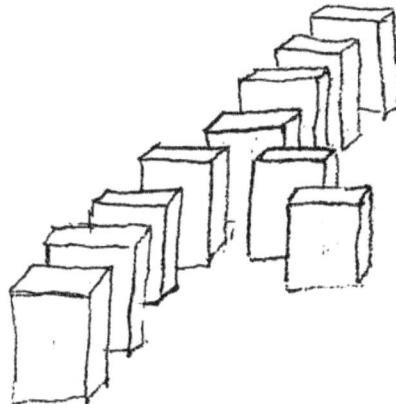

There are two types of injuries that initiate different clotting responses. Generalizing, I would call them, #1 a sharp clean razor cut and #2 a hammer blow. The differences should be pretty obvious. In the case of a the razor, blood is exposed to the same collagen fibers which activate the platelets. In the case of the hammer blow, the blood is exposed to injured tissue. (ewww... that's gross) In the injured tissue is tissue thromboplastin.

It is significant that tissue thromboplastin is outside (extrinsic) of the blood vessels and collagen is part of (intrinsic) the vasculature.

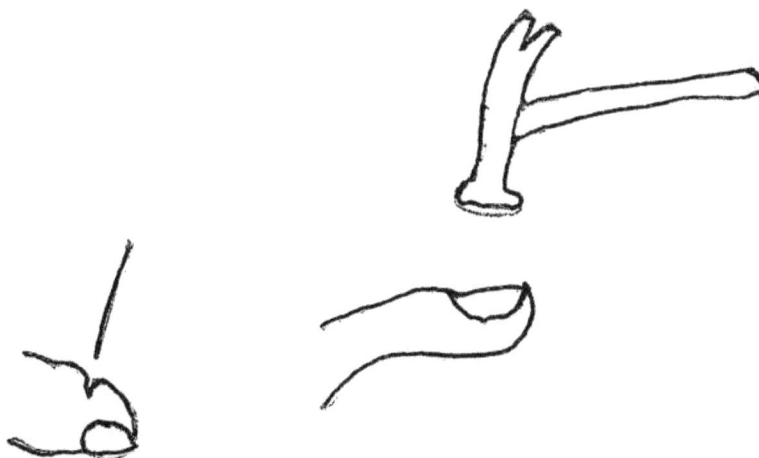

The last domino is still the same a fibrin mesh, a clot. But there are two different starting places depending on the type of injury. The sharp clean razor cut is longer path and the hammer blow is the shorter path. The more proper name is intrinsic (the razor cut) and extrinsic (the hammer blow) path.

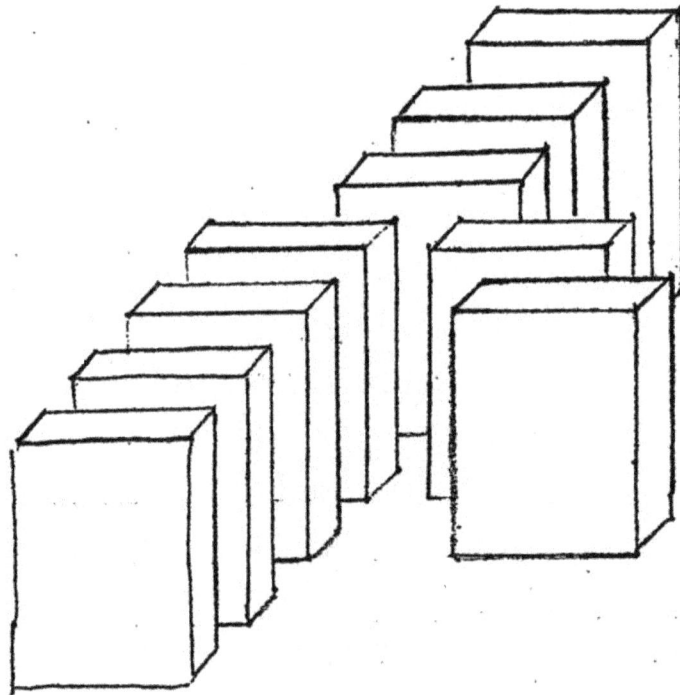

A hammer blow damages the blood vessel and exposes the blood to the damaged tissue. All tissue, your skin as an example, has a substance called tissue thromboplastin. Tissue thromboplastin activates factor VII. This sets in motion the extrinsic pathway, the shorter of the two pathways. Not only is it fewer steps, it is also less time from injury to clotting.

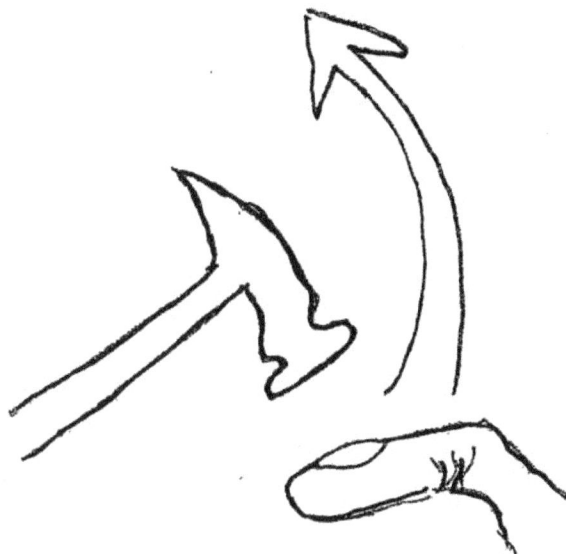

A sharp clean razor cut exposes the blood to much less injured tissue. The same exposed collagen which turned on the platelets also starts the intrinsic pathway by activation of factor XII. The number of steps (clotting factors shown as dominoes) is many more than the in extrinsic path. Perhaps you can relate to a insignificant paper cut that just keeps bleeding. Remember that sentence. It is packed with clotting facts

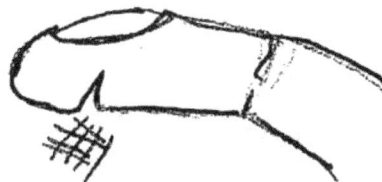

ANTITHROMBIN III and HEPARIN

The last three dominoes are called the common pathway because both the intrinsic and extrinsic pathway use the same last three clotting reactions: factor X, thrombin and fibrin. More accurately:

Inactivated factor X to activated factor X
Prothrombin to thrombin
Fibrinogen to fibrin

No matter how the clotting begins, it ends in these last three steps.

Do you remember how prostacycline stopped platelets from going crazy (aggregating) There is a similar limit to clotting: healthy endothelial cells surrounding a clot secrete antithrombin III. As the name implies, antithrombin III interferes with the conversion of prothrombin to thrombin. I have shown this as holding the domino upright or preventing it from knocking over the next domino.

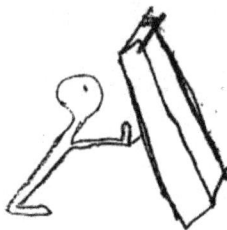

Heparin makes
 antithrombin III
four thousand (4000)
times stronger.

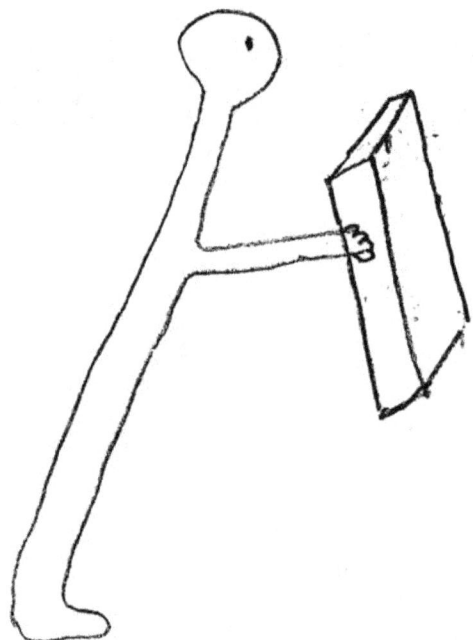

CLOT RETRACTION

Another clotting fact you may intuitively relate to is clot retraction. In the fibrin strands are actin and myocin. For a stronger clot they pull together just like muscle fiber.

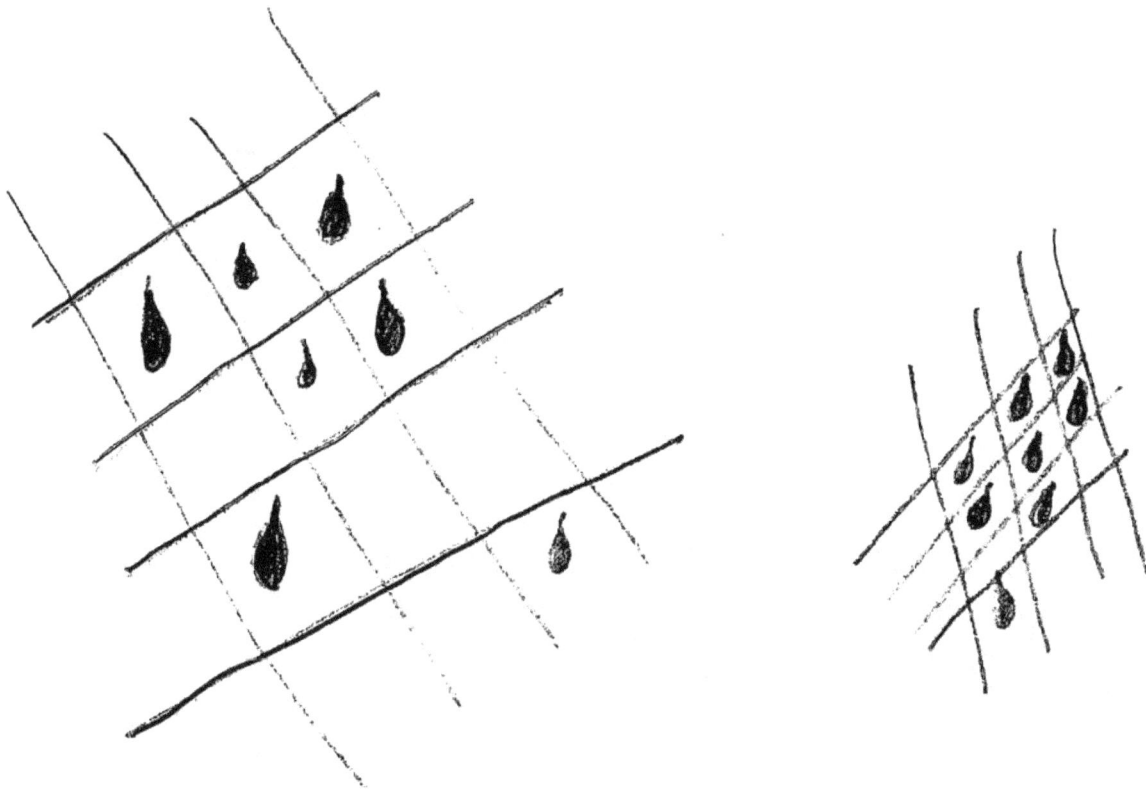

PULLING OUT A DOMINO HERE AND THERE

For the next few pages we will be looking at diseases (like hemophilia) and medications (like coumadin) which take out or put back individual clotting factors.

Let's look Hemophilia. This genetic disease is an absence of factor VIII. Missing one domino means the row cannot fall all the way to factor X and prothrombin and fibrin. Said differently, missing one domino means the row cannot fall all the way to clotting.

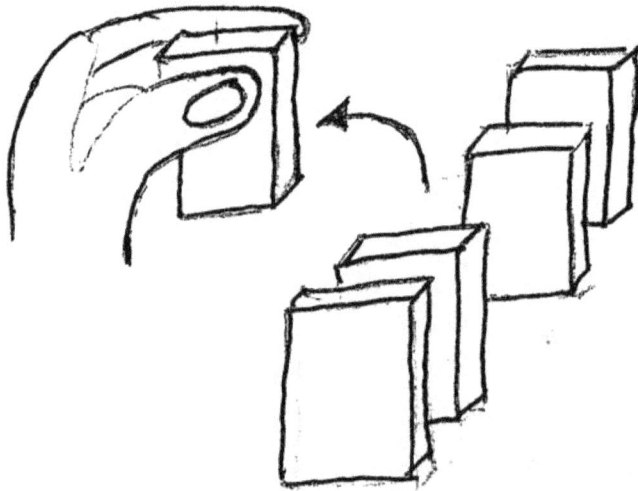

To correct this condition, plasma is given. Plasma is blood with out the red and white blood cells. Among the things left are platelets and clotting factors. So tossing in a bag (an IV bag) of clotting factors will fill in the missing space with a domino.

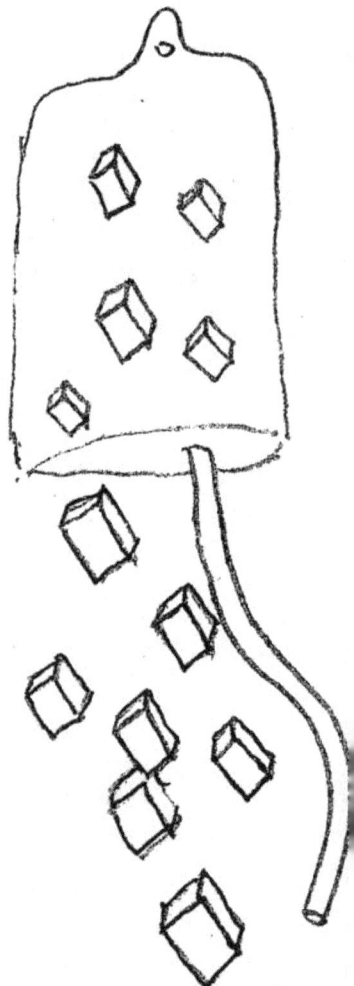

COUMADIN

You probably know coumadin is an anticoagulant. From our previous discussion you might guess that coumadin pulled out a clotting factor to slow down clotting. That would be a good first guess. What coumadin does is stop the clotting factors II, VII, IX and X from being produced. It does this by fooling the liver. Coumadin convinces the liver that it is Vitamin K. Vitamin K is essential for building those clotting factors. Less vitamin K means less clotting factors. Since coumadin has fooled the liver into thinking there is a lot of vitamin K, the liver can't produce clotting factors which depend on vitamin K.

Since coumadin stops production of factors and doesn't take them out, it takes a few days to take effect.

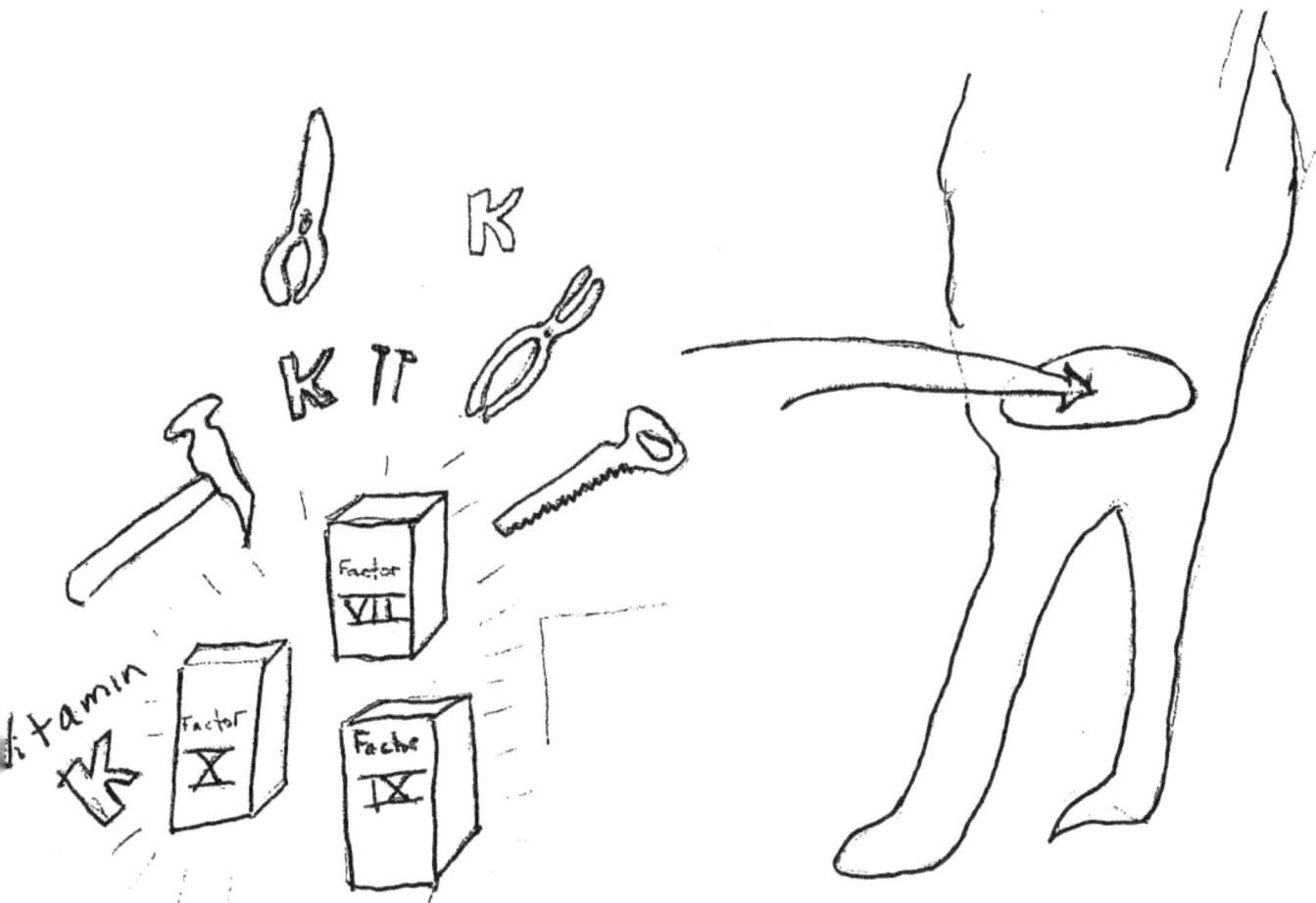

After the discussion of coumadin, it is a good time to look at another medication, Vitamin K. Vitamin K is the antidote for coumadin. Frequently prior to surgery, patients on coumadin are clotting too slowly. So as to not wait a few days for the coumadin to lose effect, vitamin K is given. If you think about what we said on the last page this makes sense. Coumadin doesn't take vitamin K out of the blood, or neutralize it. It stops the liver from producing it. So if coumadin is doing too good a job, put vitamin K back in.

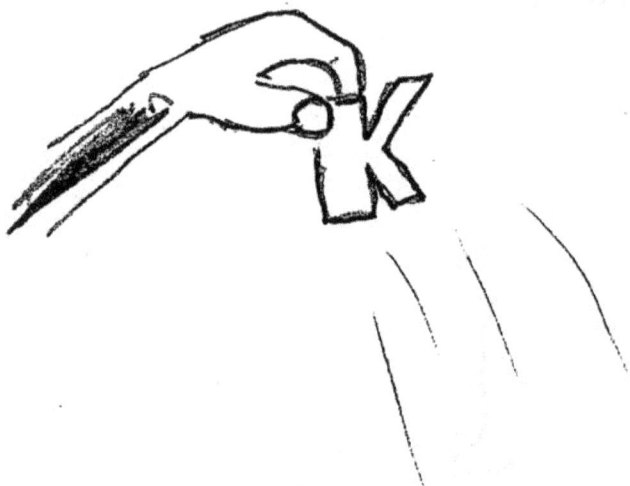

PT   PTT   INR

The prothrombin time (PT) is the length of time it takes (in seconds) for the extrinsic pathway to clot a specimen of blood. We mostly associate the PT with dosing coumadin.

There are vitamin K dependent clotting factors in the intrinsic, extrinsic and common paths. But coumadin affects factor VII in lower doses than the other vitamin K dependent factors.

The partial thromboplastin time (PTT) is the length of time for the intrinsic path to clot a specimen of blood. The extrinsic pathway is much shorter and takes less time than the intrinsic pathway.

The INR standardizes the PT. Since the PT is dependent on thromboplastin the value changes with each sample of thromboplastin. An INR would be comparable no matter where the lab got its thromboplastin.

D.I.C.
Clotting and bleeding running amok

Disseminated Intravascular Coagulation is a case where the both clotting and bleeding are out of control. D.I.C. (like ARDS) is sudden, unexpected and lethal. The name explains what it is. Disseminated means everywhere or scattered. Intravascular means within the vasculature. Coagulation means clotting. It consumes the clotting factors on a large scale.

It can be initiated by many very different causes. Among them are sepsis and tissue damage.

Because the causes are systemic, clotting appears everywhere. This is in contrast to a local clot caused by and limited to a single injury.

The end result of this wide spread coagulation is a depletion of clotting factors. I have shown this a row of fallen dominoes.

LIVER

The liver provides vitamin K which is necessary for the formation of prothrombin and factor VIII.

Vitamin K is a cofactor of clotting factor II, VII, IX, X

Vitamin K binds to calcium.

Vitamin K is the antidote to coumadin. Remember: "koumidin"

FRESH FROZEN PLASMA

Fresh frozen plasma can be found in both the frozen plasma section and the fresh plasma isle of your local blood bank.

For replacing clotting factors. In situations where the effects of coumadin have to be reversed quickly – say before emergency surgery. In the case of hemophelia where clotting factors are missing, FFP provides clotting factors.

FIBRINOLYSIS - CLOT BUSTING

As the healing of an injured vessel proceeds, removal of the clot is eventually necessary. The body accomplishes this task using plasmin, an enzyme that digests fibrin. Plasmin is produced through the activation of its precursor plasminogen. This conversion is activated by tissure plasminogen activator (TPA)

There are three drugs streptokinase, urokinase, and altepase whose therapeutic effects stem from the ability to promote conversion of plasminogen to plasmin. They are Tissue plasminogen Activators.

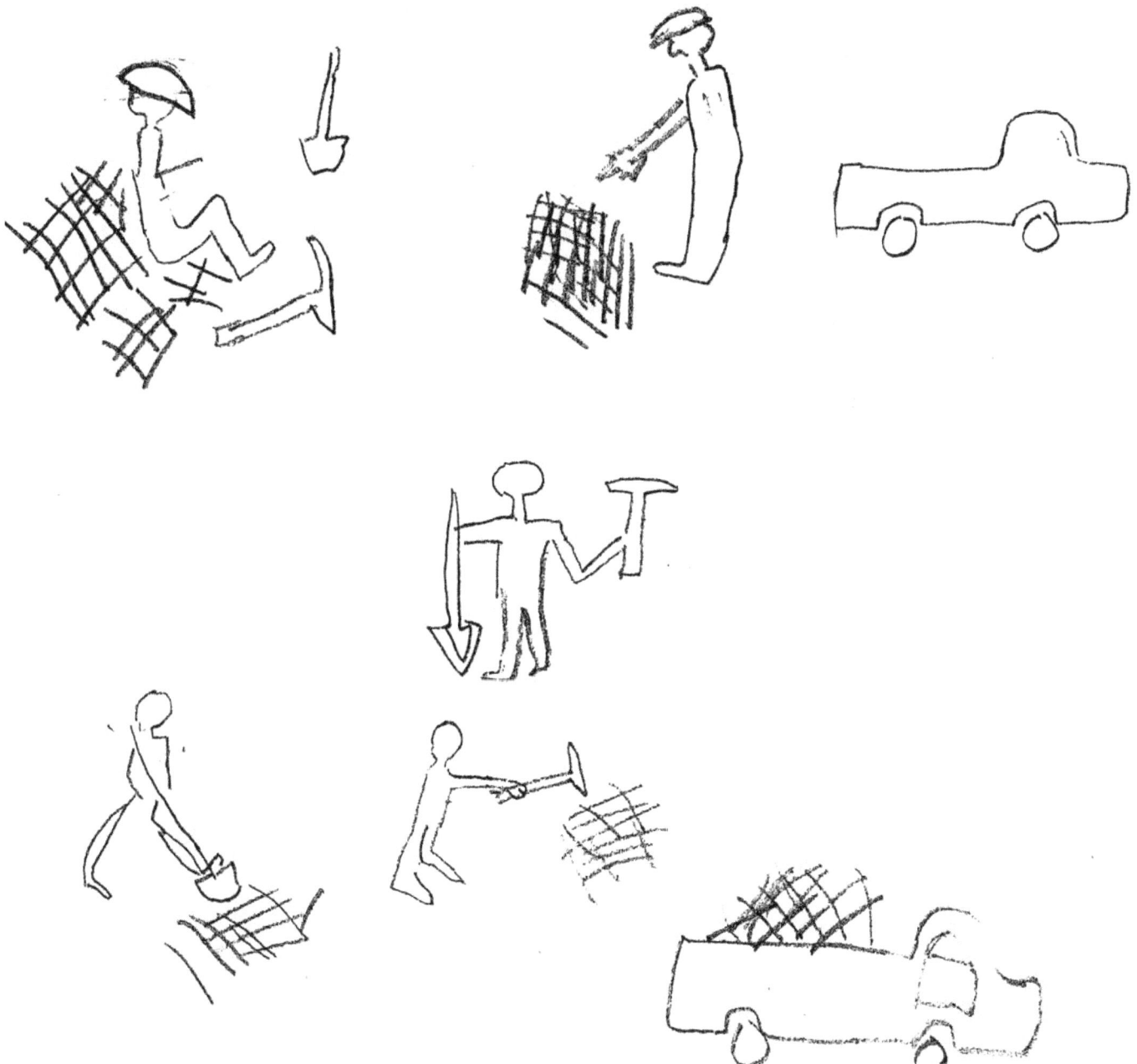

Critics call the use of drug on troops in Iraq dangerous

BY ROBERT LITTLE
BALTIMORE SUN

BAGHDAD • American military doctors in Iraq have injected more than 1,000 of the war's wounded troops with a potent and largely experimental blood-coagulating drug despite mounting medical evidence linking it to deadly blood clots that lodge in the lungs, heart and brain.

The drug, called Recombinant Activated Factor VII, is approved in the United States for treating only rare forms of hemophilia affecting about 2,700 Americans. In a warning last December, the Food and Drug Administration said that giving it to patients with normal blood could cause strokes and heart attacks. Its researchers published a study in January blaming 43 deaths on clots that developed after injections of Factor VII.

The U.S. Army medical command considers Factor VII to be a medical breakthrough in the war, giving frontline physicians a powerful new means of controlling bleeding that can be treated otherwise only with surgery and transfusions. They have posted guidelines at military field hospitals encouraging its liberal use in all casualties with severe bleeding, and doctors in Iraq routinely inject it into patients upon the mere anticipation of deadly bleeding to come.

"When it works, it's amazing," said Col. John B. Holcomb, an Army trauma surgeon and the service's top adviser on combat medical care. "It's one of the most useful new tools we have."

Yet the Army's faith in the $6,000-a-dose drug is based almost entirely on anecdotal evidence and persists despite public warnings and published research suggesting that Factor VII is not as effective or as safe as military officials say.

Doctors and researchers at

considering reports from military doctors in Iraq describing its success at controlling severe bleeding.

"I've seen it with my own eyes," said Air Force Lt. Col. Jeffrey Bailey, a trauma surgeon deployed this summer as senior physician at the American military hospital in Balad, Iraq. "Patients who are hemorrhaging to death, they get the drug and it stops. Factor VII saves their lives."

Military officials are unapologetic about moving aggressively toward a new treatment for the types of deadly bleeding they see frequently in Iraq. Wounded troops requiring transfusions of 10 or more units of blood have a 25 percent to 50 percent chance of dying from their injuries, they say.

"We're making decisions, in the middle of a war, with the best information we have available to us," said Holcomb, commander of the Army's Institute of Surgical Research. "We're not waiting" for more clinical research, he said.

As the trauma adviser to the Army surgeon general, it was Holcomb's decision, with the support of Army leadership, to begin using Factor VII as a standard treatment in Iraq.

The Baltimore Sun is a Tribune Co. newspaper.

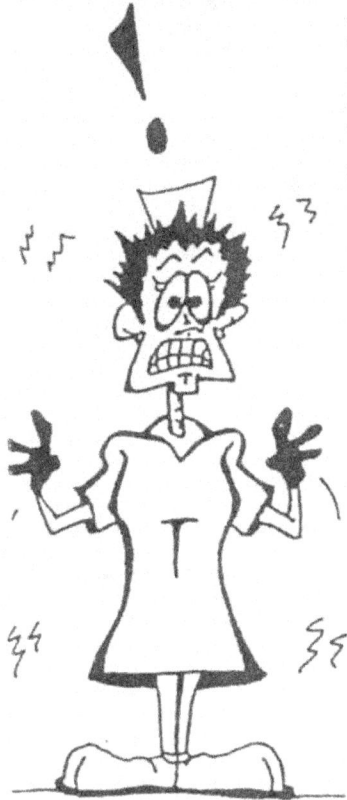
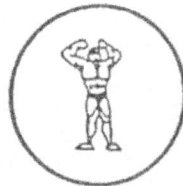
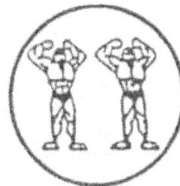
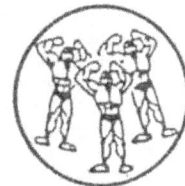
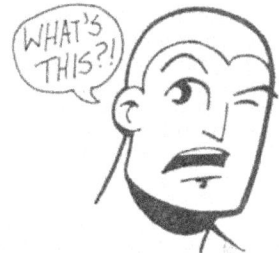
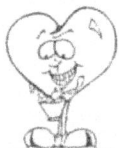
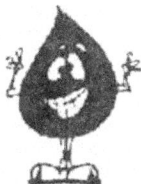
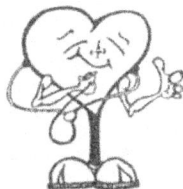
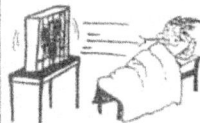
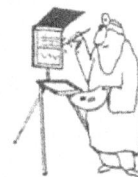
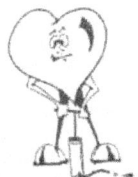

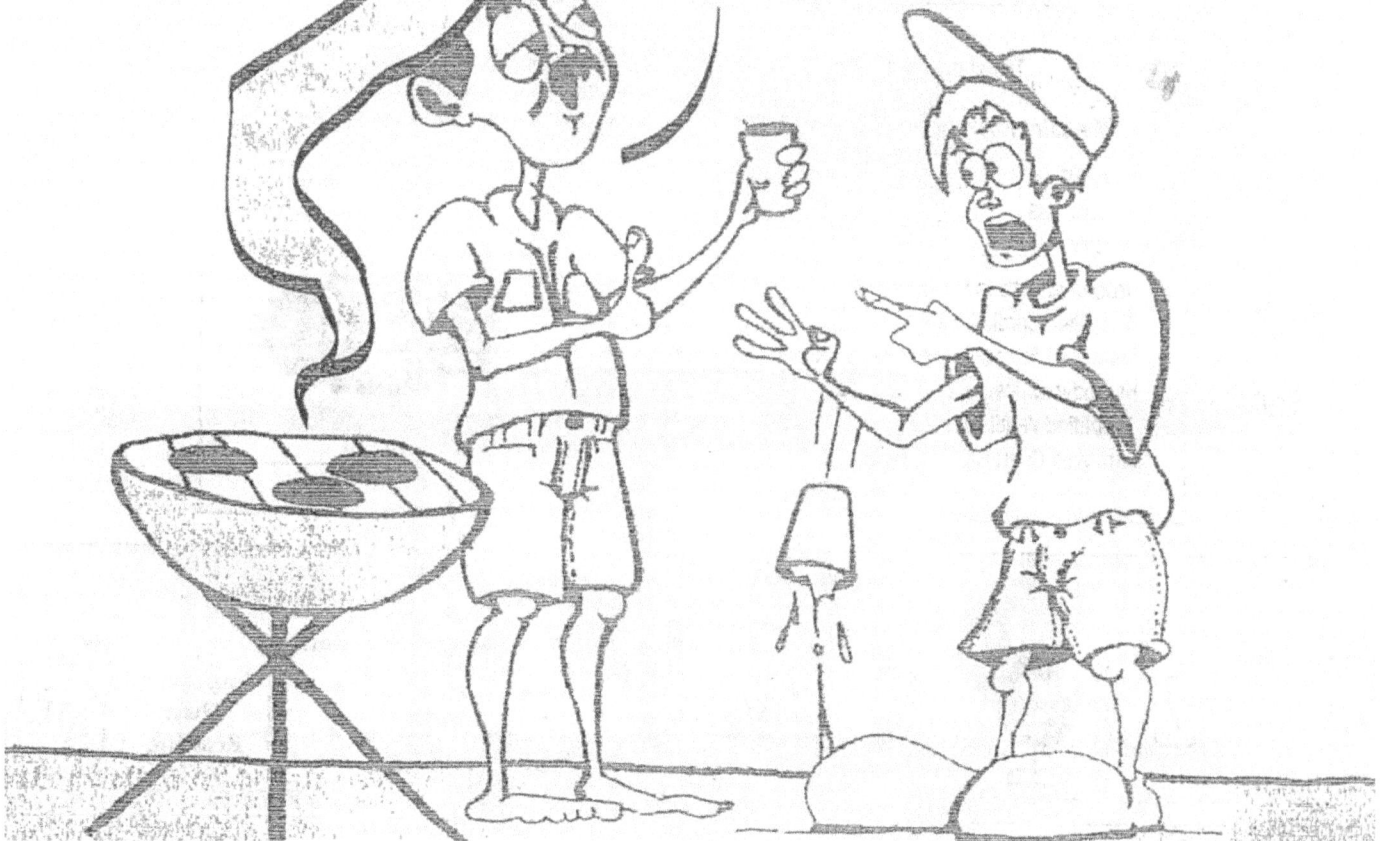

Simplified Clotting ©2007

Retail: $7.95

ISBN 0-9725483-6-X

9780972548366

0 700814 498054

7 00814 49805 4